Sheng Zhen

Awakening the Soul

A FORM OF SHENG ZHEN GONG
THE QIGONG OF UNCONDITIONAL LOVE

WITH

Master Li Junfeng

PUBLISHED BY
THE INTERNATIONAL SHENG ZHEN SOCIETY FOUNDATION, INC.

www.shengzhen.org

THE ISZS FOUNDATION

The International Sheng Zhen Society Foundation is a non-profit organization which had its beginnings in 1995. It was formed to promote the spirit of Sheng Zhen – the spirit of unconditional love, through propagating the Sheng Zhen practices throughout the world. Through the commitment of those who believe and want to help in this loving mission, books, audio recordings and videos, have been produced to enable practitioners to study the Sheng Zhen forms, teachings and philosophy. The ISZS Foundation has also made it possible for Li Junfeng, its head and principal teacher, to travel around the world teaching students, training teachers and planting seeds of love so that this vision to create a world steeped in unconditional love becomes a reality.

To date there are certified teachers and practitioners in key locations in the USA, Canada, Europe, Africa, Australia, New Zealand, and Asia.

For more information on classes and workshops we invite you to visit: www.shengzhen.org

NOTE ON THE TEXT

Allow yourself to read what is written here free of fixed concepts attached to the words "soul", "spirit", and "heart". To explain the practice of Awakening the Soul, we use these words in an expanded way in order to describe what takes place in this form of timeless and universal healing.

Contents

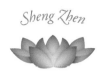

FOREWORD

In an Increasingly Complex World that demands much from an individual, it is reassuring to know that there exist practices supported by philosophies that have the power to bring an experience of harmony, purpose, and ease back to the challenging life on this planet. Many true spiritual paths have the power to do this.

One such philosophy and way of life is Sheng Zhen (pronounced shung jen) – translated as sacred truth, the highest truth, which is unconditional love. The beauty of this philosophy, that teaches that everything comes from love and goes back to love, is the manner in which the learning and the transformation takes place. The philosophy is articulated and experienced through moving and non-moving forms of qigong, accompanied by messages or contemplations. At the onset, the practices may appear like beautiful movements that could be seen as physical exercise, similar to dance. The non-moving forms bring much needed relaxation to weary minds and stressful lives. Like most forms of beneficial qigong, it is good for the physical health, the mind, and the emotions.

The Sheng Zhen system of practices and its philosophy* takes another step. Like other forms of qigong, blockages lodged in the body, the mind, and the emotions causing various disorders are gradually removed, bringing about a sense of wellness. However, it doesn't stop here. Very naturally, the practitioner begins to experience the opening of the heart. A heart that is open is the foundation of true wellness. It is the place from which relationships are healed and good ones develop. It is the seat of wisdom and understanding. A sense of purpose is born from an open heart. This is where compassion develops – compassion for oneself and for others. A feeling of connectedness to the planet and to the entire universe can only happen in an open heart. How one experiences the heart determines the quality of one's life.

When the heart is open, not only does love reside in it, one lives in love. It is not simply that you carry the experience of perfection and fullness within the heart; you actually begin to see perfection everywhere. This happens at a natural pace; an awakening can happen as instantly as waking up from a dream or as gradually as fruit ripening on a tree.

At the very least, the Sheng Zhen practices have the power to make one feel physically better, become happier, more relaxed and at ease with oneself and one's surroundings. Whatever you wish to take away from the practices is yours. You can approach it from any level. It is a compassionate system that calibrates itself to you. You may be happy to just dip your toe into the ocean of love that is offered. You may want to immerse yourself in that ocean. Or you may want to experience that you are the ocean of love – infinitely deep and expansive. This form of gigong called Awakening the Soul is for those new to Sheng Zhen, as well as for those who have more experience.

Looking back at the more than twelve years I have been doing the Sheng Zhen practices I have seen my respect and appreciation for the gifts of Sheng Zhen deepen as time passes. I have seen old destructive habits (both physical and mental) dissolve and be replaced by a sense of openness and balance. I have a much better understanding of my body and how it affects my mind and my inner state and vice versa. I have seen how others have been transformed by the power inherent to the practices. It is truly a humbling experience to watch and be a part of this amazing process within myself and in others. For many years I had the good fortune of living close by to our beloved Teacher Li, our qigong master who brought these practices into our lives. We now live half a world apart and the Sheng Zhen family of practitioners is now everywhere, spanning the globe. In a way, the physical distance makes it more apparent that we are one in the heart, making the world a more intimate, loving place.

May this practice called Awakening the Soul answer our deepest yearnings. May it bring all of us back to the freshness of a new beginning where all becomes possible once again. May our lives become an expression of the inner joy which is our essence. May the experience we gain from Awakening the Soul add to the ever-expanding world of the heart, the place where all answers are found, and lasting fulfilment and true freedom is experienced.

- Anabel Alejandrino

To further deepen your understanding, you may want to consult the book, Sheng Zhen Wuji Yuan Gong, A Return to Oneness, view the video DVD set, or seek further instruction from a certified Sheng Zhen teacher.

INTRODUCTION

The Soul is the Vehicle of the Spirit on this Realm. The soul mirrors the spirit. The clarity of the soul reflects the stillness of the spirit. Quality of life on this realm is determined by the state of the soul and spirit upon coming into this realm. . . as well as the choices one makes in life.

The soul may also be understood and examined in relation to the heart. What is the heart? Aside from the physical heart itself, it is, what we may call, the individual's subjective principle, i.e., temperament, emotions, attitude, state of mind. An individual's soul may also be seen as part of the heart. The heart is connected to the spirit through the soul. Being its vehicle, the spirit functions on this realm through the soul, through the heart. An individual's health, his moral character and his understanding of life is linked to how he is in touch with his heart and soul.

It is possible to reconnect with one's original state at birth. Through the practice of Awakening the Soul, one is able to return to the beginning, return to the newness of coming into this realm for the first time. When the soul is awakened, the experience is like breathing new life into the body. The key to awakening the soul is the opening of the heart.

When the heart is open, it possesses the qualities of willingness and suppleness, of having a natural sense of wonder and freedom from fear. As these qualities grow and develop, as the heart opens, one can return to the origin, to breathe the original breath and become one with the pulse of the universe. This gigong, called Awakening the Soul, has the power to achieve this. Upon reaching this state, when the soul is awakened, one's life becomes inspired, and doubt and worry cease to exist. The burden of life becomes non-existent as in a newborn child. Then, one's own awakened soul, one's open heart, becomes the doorway to freedom and clarity.

Awakening the Soul also means distilling the soul, clarifying the soul. With renewed clarity, one gains a deeper understanding of one's life and what truly matters. It becomes clear that the experience of unconditional love is the most valuable thing one can attain in life. To experience the heart at its fullest, one must cultivate love. The soil of the heart must be tilled to harvest the sweet fruit of unconditional love. In living by this truth, one learns how to enjoy life. Being happy comes naturally. What follows is a sense of perfect well-being, a sense of profound contentment.

Through the practice of Awakening the Soul, may all people experience the opening of the heart, the freshness of returning to the beginning, and the simplicity of once again becoming one with nature and the universe. Then, all can experience true love, understand life, and enjoy life fully – body and soul!

Awakening the Soul
&
Sheng Zhen

The Movements of Awakening the Soul are easy to learn. This qigong is the most basic qigong within the Sheng Zhen Gong system. It leads naturally into Sheng Zhen Gong proper. It serves as a guide to life, a gift given at the start of the spiritual journey. It is the stepping-stone towards the final goal. It can lead people into the sweetest and the most beautiful state that is the gift of Sheng Zhen Gong.

It is our hope that those who learn Awakening the Soul move into the practice of the Union of Three Hearts Meditation and eventually go into the moving forms that comprise Sheng Zhen Gong. This is the purpose of Awakening the Soul – to draw people into the deeper Sheng Zhen practices.

The movements of Sheng Zhen Gong are unique and unparalleled. May those who eventually become practitioners of Sheng Zhen Gong explore and discover its inner beauty. Although the physical movements are beautiful, to experience its inner as well as its outer beauty – its perfection, is the goal of the practice.

The purpose and philosophy of Sheng Zhen Gong hold the highest teachings. It is important for the practitioner to understand the Sheng Zhen mission – that all of humanity experience peace and oneness, and harmony with nature; to help humanity in discovering life's purpose. Through this mission's work, it becomes possible to attain a fulfilling life – to be healthier, happier. Through the mission, one is gifted with a more positive attitude, capable of embracing the ups and downs of life. The warm smile of a heart that is filled with love and joy invokes blessings to the entire world. This is the mission of Sheng Zhen and this is the motivation for your practice – to transform the peace and happiness in every person's heart to become the collective heart of a humankind immersed in love.

ZHONGTIAN MOVEMENT

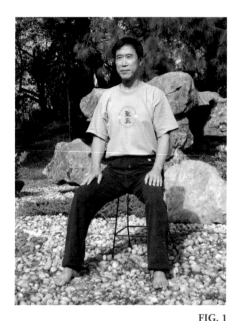

FIG. 1

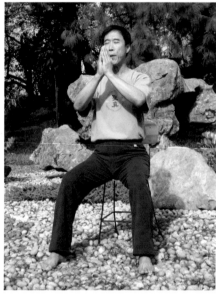

FIG. 2

THE ZHONGTIAN MOVEMENT *symbolizes the cleansing of the hands, face and heart. Its deeper meaning is to connect to heaven and earth and to merge with the universe. You feel your body is pure and one with the universe.*

Every form of Sheng Zhen Gong begins and ends with the Zhongtian Movement.

1. Sit comfortably on the edge of a chair with feet flat on floor. Rest palms on top of thighs (**FIG. 1**).

Raise both hands; bring them together with palms facing each other. Hands are slightly cupped with thumbs apart while tips of other fingers and outer edges of hands touch (**FIG. 2**). Gently blow into the space between palms.

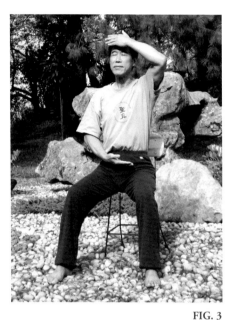

| FIG. 3 | FIG. 4 |

2. Separate hands; move right hand down to slightly below navel and simultaneously move left hand up to sweep across the front of the face from chin to forehead (**FIG. 3**). Continue to move left hand, sweeping it downward in front of face and torso until it comes to rest on palm of right hand.

3. Arms are bent slightly at the elbows; upper arms are held slightly away from torso. The palms of the hands face up and the tips of thumbs touch forming a heart-shaped hollow space (**FIG. 4**).

FIRST MOVEMENT
Opening the Heart

In the core of the soul that yearns to be free

Shines the light of a gentle moonbeam

Piercing the daunting darkness of illusion

Lightly caressing the heart open to see

A sky so clear, air so refreshing

It is so familiar though still a memory

Questions arise. What lies beyond?

Is it just a moonbeam? Will it stay a wish?

Nourished by intention blessed by sweet effort

With a little bit of faith and a pure sense of wonder

Ever so gently ever so slowly

The moon of the heart is revealed

FIRST MOVEMENT

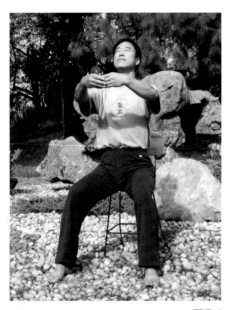

FIG. 5

FIG. 6

PREPARATION:

Quiet your mind; relax your body; feel the qi from your body expand. You are merged with the universe. You are one with the universe.

1. While inhaling, slowly raise both arms **(FIG. 5)**. When hands reach higher than chest level, gradually open hands diagonally outwards and upwards, until head level or a little higher. Palms facing body, wrists are relaxed. At the same time, lean back slightly, tilting head back naturally; turn up toes and rest feet on heels **(FIG. 6)**.

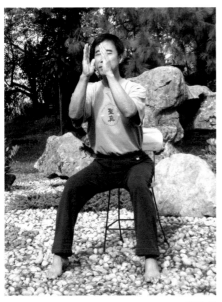

FIG. 7

FIG. 8

2. While exhaling, allow body weight to shift slightly forward, moving hands inward so both palms face each other. Bring palms towards each other until they are about head-width apart, at face level, while raising heels (**FIG. 7**). The head and torso are in line. Naturally contract the chest and relax. Prepare to open again.

3. While inhaling, shift body weight slightly back, the head and hands gradually get farther away from each other, as you open the arms; let the upper arms lead the lower arms and hands. Hands move diagonally outwards, until head level or a littler higher. Turn up toes and rest feet on heels (**FIG. 8**).

4. Exhale and repeat directions in 2.

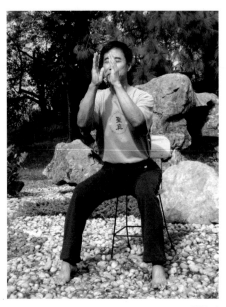

FIG. 9   **FIG. 10**

5. Repeat many times (**FIG. 9, 10**).

POINTS TO REMEMBER:

A. *Synchronize body movement with the breath. Breathe deeply from the chest. When you inhale and open your arms, imagine the chest is open and expanding to the universe. The more relaxed the breathing, the slower the movement.*

B. *The movement of the arms must be continuous. The level of the hands may be higher or lower.*

C. *Always remember to smile and enjoy the movements. Forget yourself. Think only of the movement. Expand the chest and allow the heart to open so that the body, heart, and mind merge with the universe.*

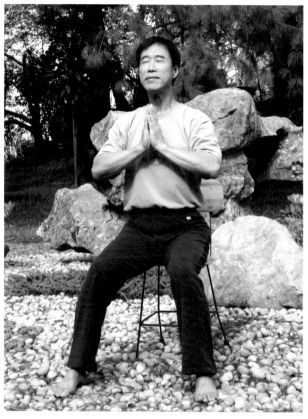

D. *The movement of body and feet are synchronized. The feet shift from toe to heel as the body rocks forward and backward.*
E. *The number of repetitions depends on one's level of comfort. Breathe from the chest.*

FIG. 11

6. To finish, exhale, the body becomes erect and hands come closer, ending in prayer position at the heart (**FIG. 11**).

17

SECOND MOVEMENT

Love Descends on Me

Like a trusting child at the moment of birth

I receive the love that descends

I am bathed in the nourishing kindness of qi

I believe in the gifts of the universe

The moonbeam is now a sure shaft of light

That stills the chatter of my doubting mind

I revel in the love that embraces me

I am safe I am fearless I know I am ready

May the Heavens guard the opening of my heart

To see the clarity that is my core

In that knowledge is my courage

In that strength lies even more

SECOND MOVEMENT

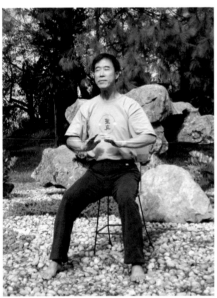 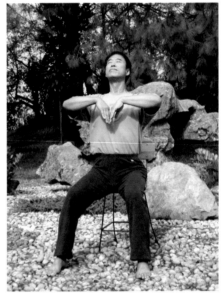

FIG. 12

FIG. 13

1. Exhale. Naturally relax the body. Allow hands to go down and gradually separate heels of hands (**FIG. 12**).

2. Inhale. Straighten the body. Raising upper arms, hands follow and move upwards; backs of fingers gently touch. Wrists are relaxed. (**FIG. 13**).

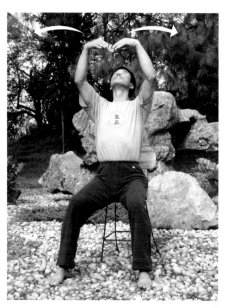

FIG. 14

FIG. 15

3. Continue to raise hands above the head (**FIG. 14**), slightly raising chin while gradually opening the arms towards sides, wrists becoming straight and palms face upwards; fingers are naturally separated. Hold arms at about face level as long as you can (**FIG. 15**).

POINTS TO REMEMBER:

A. *If you do not have the physical strength to hold the arms up, it is enough to imagine doing so.*

B. *Imagine your body and hands open to the universe to invite more qi and love into the body.*

C. *In order to relax your body more and stimulate a greater flow of qi you may repeat movements in* **FIGS. 12-13** *several times before proceeding to* **FIG. 14**.

THIRD MOVEMENT
Unravelling the Heart

The knot in the heart is the feeling of smallness

That we know as fear, shame, or pain

It is slowly unravelled so gently undone,

Setting the heart free to move once again

In the silence of the process beneath the feelings
of smallness

Within lies a wealth we find and revealed

Our own understanding compassion for ourselves

The foundation of a heart that is healed

Relax and listen to the stirrings of the heart

Be ready for that wave of recall

When we delight in the pleasure in the knowledge
and treasure

The freshness, the awakening of the soul

THIRD MOVEMENT

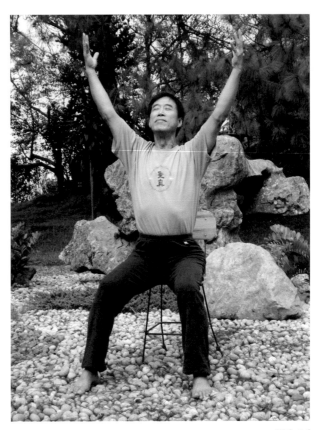

FIG. 16

1. Gradually raise arms and move hands in an arc upward towards each other (**FIG. 16**).

Unravelling the Heart

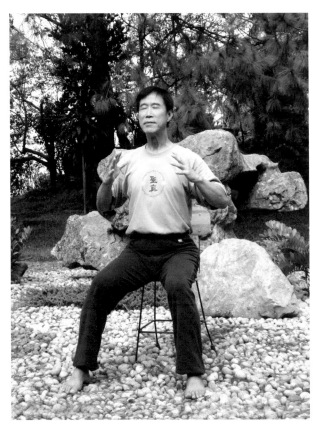

FIG. 17

POINTS TO
REMEMBER:

A. *Keep body and
head upright to feel the
chest expand and open.
Slightly arch the back.*
B. *Keep the shoulders
relaxed while leaving
some space between the
arms and torso.*
C. *Keep the arms in
line from fingertips to
elbow. Do not bend or
flex the wrists.*
D. *Fingers are naturally
extended and spread
apart but relaxed.*

2. Let arms gradually descend so hands end
up in front of chest about head-width apart
or a little wider (**FIG. 17**). Hold this position for
some time.

FOURTH MOVEMENT
Suddenly Lifting the Veil

In an instant it happens the heart knows the song

The soul knows the dance of the full moon's

   moonlight

Suddenly it comes the freedom of knowing

Of basking in the joy of now remembering

The weight of exertion is lifted away

The illusion of weariness dissolved by the moonlight

No longer just a memory much more than familiar

That light seen at birth that is now here to stay

Fearlessness, freedom, fullness of being

The inner delight of simply existing

The purity, the clarity, the bliss of recalling

The awakening of the soul, a brand new beginning!

FOURTH MOVEMENT

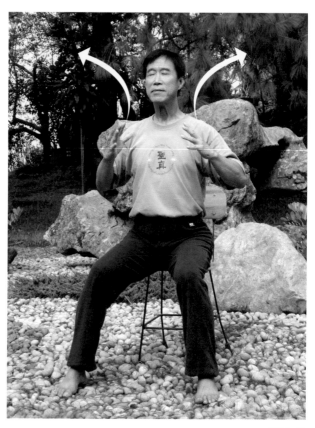

FIG. 18

1. While arching the spine, lift the chin, bring elbows closer and move hands apart. Hands diagonally point up, out and forwards, opening the chest **(FIG. 18-19)**.

Suddenly Lifting the Veil

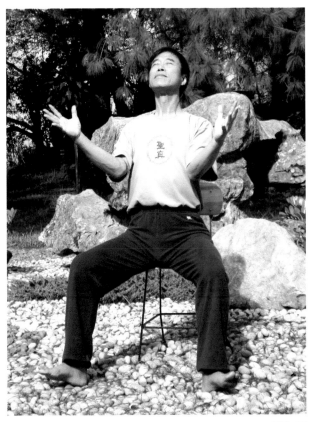

FIG. 19

POINTS TO
REMEMBER:
*Feel that your heart
and body are completely
open. You are happy
and content.*

2. With some force, extend and separate fingers while slightly leaning back. At the same time, move thighs apart, lift toes, pointing them outwards. Hold for some time (**FIG. 19**).

FIFTH MOVEMENT

Holding the Heavens
Grounded on Earth

A luminous space with an endless sky

Welcoming one to the moment of dawning

All smallness dissolves in the mighty expansion

There are no boundaries to this new beginning

A world is shown of infinite possibilities

Lovingly offered to one unconditionally

Confidence, openness, a new sense of being

There is strength to embrace all that can be

Rooted in life yet holding the universe

Being and non-being immersed in believing

Receiving the gift to once again see

I know I am light I yearn to be free

FIFTH MOVEMENT

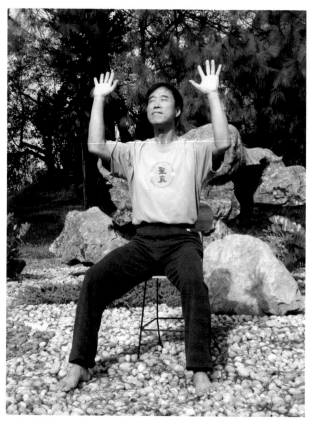

FIG. 20

1. Gradually move hands backwards and upwards, rotating them inwards, opening elbows. Feet return to previous position **(FIG. 20)**.

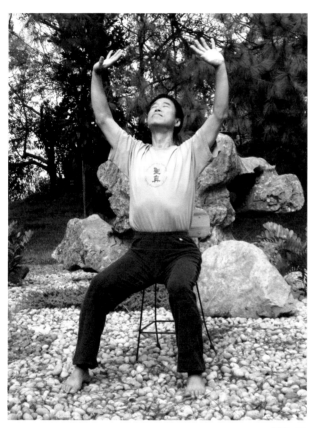

FIG. 21

2. Continue to rotate hands, extend arms up
and hands push with some force. Palms face up,
fingers separated almost pointing to each other,
elbows slightly bent. Keep chin naturally lifted.
Hold this position **(FIG. 21)**.

SIXTH MOVEMENT
Freeing Oneself to Become a Saint

Where does one go from this point on?

Is it simply existence with no boundaries?

Is there more to know to be and to see?

How does one grasp what it means to be free?

Tasting the experience leads to understanding

That receiving the gift requires something more

One needs to practice to keep the heart open

To become rooted in the bliss at the core

When the soul is awakened there is one true desire

To become one in the heart with no restraint

This giving of oneself with no conditions

Is freeing oneself to become a saint

SIXTH MOVEMENT

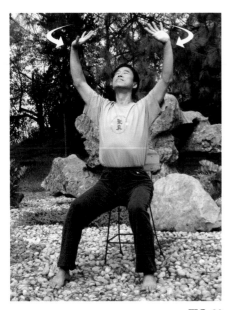

FIG. 22

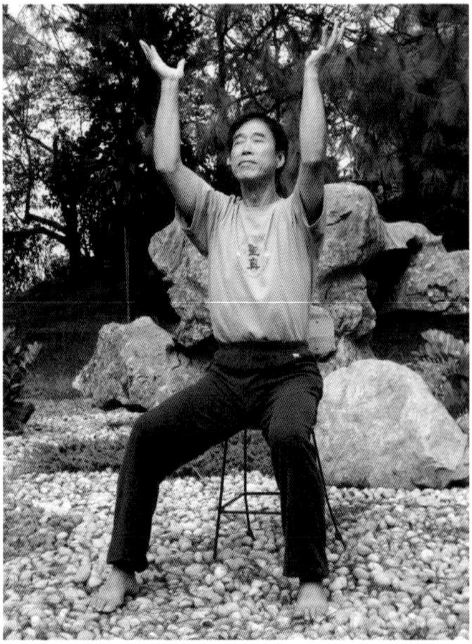

FIG. 23

1. Move elbows inwards rotating hands **(FIG. 22)**, gradually lowering them.

2. Bring heels of the hands together in front of chest **(FIG. 23)**.

Freeing Oneself to Become a Saint

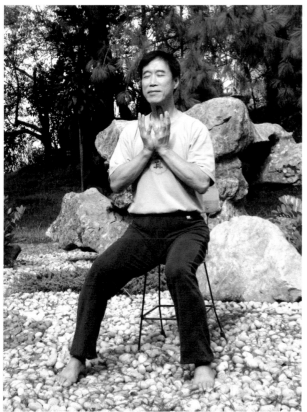

FIG. 24

POINTS TO
REMEMBER:
A. *Heels of hands,
thumbs, and small
fingers touch without
excess pressure.*
B. *Bringing elbows
slightly inward will
allow fingers to relax
more easily.*

3. Thumbs and small fingers touch, other
fingers are spread apart, like a lotus flower.
Hold this position (**FIG. 24**).

SEVENTH MOVEMENT

Walk to the Center of Heaven

The lotus of the heart is now in full bloom

Through the tunnel of light it glows, it rises

The crescendo of love swells to the crown

Echoing, expanding like waves in the ocean

I walk into that space I walk into that state

It now has become much more than just fate

Light upon light revealing the splendor

The moment before birth in Heaven's Center

In the infinite pause beyond the threshold of time

Is the doorway for souls that dive into life

And at the end of a life of a heart that is open

Is the very same doorway to the Center of Heaven

SEVENTH MOVEMENT

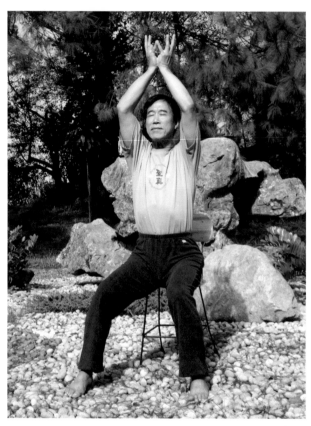

FIG. 25

1. While inhaling, slowly raise hands higher than head (**FIG. 25**).

Walk to the Center of Heaven

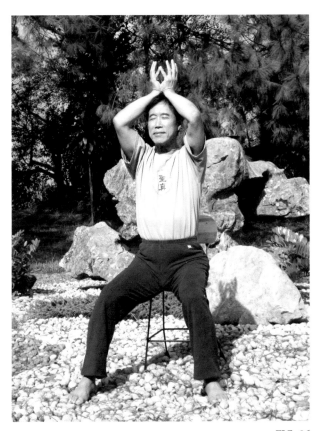

FIG. 26

2. Exhaling, bring hands slightly backward and slowly downward. Rest base of hands gently on top of the crown of the head. Hold this position (**FIG. 26**).

EIGHTH MOVEMENT
Return to the Origin

A thirst of the heart, all forms of yearning

Is a longing to return to the point of origin

A desire to reclaim the Self long forgotten

To taste the deep contentment of just simply being

Like the ongoing cycle of birth and death

The natural sequence of hold and release

The flow of the in breath the flow of the out breath

The circle is completed with the simplest of ease

The surrender that gives into the womb of
    nothingness

Becomes everything and nothing at all

There is only consciousness, a deep profound stillness

The seamless silence that is both empty and full

EIGHTH MOVEMENT

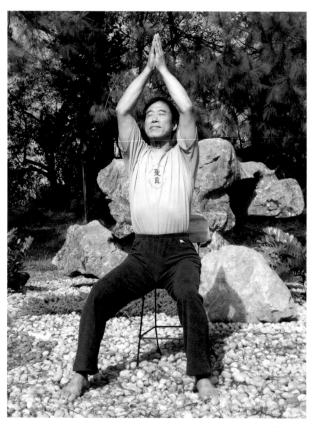

FIG. 27

1. Naturally raise hands, palms gradually come together **(FIG. 27)**.

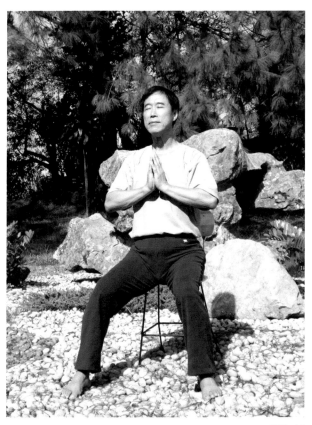

FIG. 28

2. Lower hands to prayer position at
the heart (**FIG. 28**). Hold for a long time.
Think of nothing. Return to nothingness.

CLOSING MOVEMENT

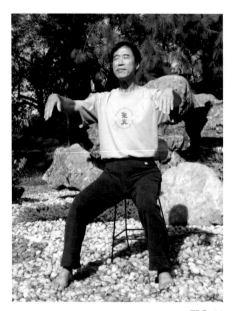

FIG. 29

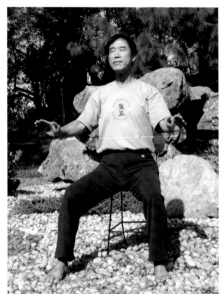

FIG. 30

1. To end, while inhaling, relax hands and separate them to shoulder-width apart (**FIG. 29**).

2. Exhale and drop elbows (**FIG. 30**).

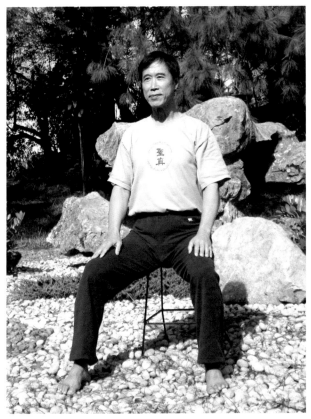

FIG. 31

3. Allow arms to fall until hands rest with palms down on thighs (**FIG. 31**).

In closing, do the **Zhongtian Movement** as on pages 10-11.

About Master Li

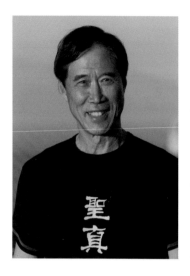

Master Li Junfeng is the principal teacher and head of the International Sheng Zhen Society. He is the moving force behind bringing Sheng Zhen Gong, the Qigong of Unconditional Love to the world. His life and his way of being are a living testament to the teachings embodied in this loving form of qigong. Teacher Li, as he is affectionately called, is a master of qigong who emphasizes both the physical and spiritual aspects of this practice. Sheng Zhen Gong is not only good for the emotional and physical body, but also opens the heart, and elevates one's spirit.

Master Li is perhaps best known as having been the national team coach for the women's division of the world-renowned Beijing Wushu (Martial Arts) Team of the People's Republic of China. For over twelve years, under his leadership, individual students won nearly 100 gold medals in national and international competitions, elevating the standards of excellence worldwide. During his coaching years, he also achieved international fame as a martial arts film actor and choreographer.

Master Li travels to train Sheng Zhen Gong teachers, to practice with his students, and to simply spend time with them. In so doing he shares his wisdom, his understanding, his love – his entire being, so that others too may experience the joy and contentment that permeate his life. Simply being with him enables one to grasp and experience the depth and the beauty of this loving practice.

May the practice of Awakening the Soul answer
our deepest yearnings.

May it bring all of us back to the freshness of a
new beginning where all becomes possible once again.

May our lives become an expression of the inner joy
that is our very essence.

May the experience we gain from Awakening the
Soul add to the ever-expanding world of the heart,
the place where all answers are found and lasting
fulfilment and true freedom are experienced.

Sheng Zhen

Sheng Zhen

Sheng Zhen